NO! NO! NO!

NO!
NO!
NO!

*A Woman's Guide
to Personal Defense
and Street Safety*

KATHY LONG
WITH DAVIS MILLER

Photographs by Pete Conteras and Eric Nolan

A PERIGEE BOOK

Perigee Books
are published by
The Putnam Publishing Group
200 Madison Avenue
New York, NY 10016

Library of Congress Cataloging-in-Publication Data

Long, Kathy.
    NO! NO! NO! : a woman's guide to personal defense and
street safety / by Kathy Long with Davis Miller ; photographs
by Pete Conteras.
      p.   cm.
    ISBN 0-399-51845-2
    1. Self-defense for women. I. Miller, Davis. II. Title.
GV1111.5.L66 1993   93-26754 CIP
613.6'6—dc20

Cover design by Isabella Fasciano
Cover photo © 1993 by Buddy Rosenberg

Printed in the United States of America
1 2 3 4 5 6 7 8 9 10

The authors wish to thank: Laura Shepherd, Peter Nelson, Alison B. Cranford, Michael Turner, Jimmy Vasquez, Rob Irwin, the National Victim Center, and the Crime Victims Research and Treatment Center.

To Eric, the source and the inspiration.
— KL

To Lynn, for hanging in there.
— DM

Contents

NO! NO! NO!

Introduction

WHAT ARE THE REALITIES?

According to FBI statistics, more than seventy percent of women in America encounter violent crime within their lifetimes. One out of every eight women currently living in the United States has been a rape victim. Eighty-three percent of all rape victims are women under twenty-five years of age. Every hour, seventy-eight women in the United States report that they have been raped. Each day, roughly 3,000 report that they have been victims of some form of forced aggression. These, of course, are the reported occurrences. Far more sexual (and nonsexual) assaults go unreported.

You are in danger. And you need to be prepared—not just physically, but emotionally. Often, on television and in movies, when a female character tries to escape an attacker, she doesn't even know how to run. We see her twisting an ankle as she attempts to escape in high heels or, if she's wearing flats, stumbling along in a prissy, spasmodic manner that looks as if she's absolutely incapable. The cultural message, the intimation, is that you are helpless. The reality, of course, is that you're not.

If you are attacked and decide to fight back, the techniques in this manual can work for you. But this does not necessarily mean that they will.

I have taught hundreds of women how to defend themselves. Most of those people who *wanted* to become capable of defending themselves were able to do so. They became street-smart and have been successful when they needed to be.

I don't want you to think, though, that I offer any magic martial art that will make you impervious to harm. Most martial arts books and classes tend to give a false sense of power, make you feel you can thwart would-be attackers with relative ease. It's essential from the outset that you understand the realities.

One of the first things you need to know is that you may need to change your basic mind-set about personal defense and about the ways in which the world works. We live in an increasingly dangerous time. In contemporary America, it's best to develop a little healthy paranoia. You don't have a protective bubble around you; you can't count on a guardian angel or some other supernatural force protecting you. It's imperative that you recognize that, at all times, everywhere, you may be attacked, mugged, assaulted, raped, and killed. You are every bit as vulnerable as the victims you read about in your newspaper.

It helps to know your chances. And to know where violent and nonviolent crimes against women are most likely to take place. In later chapters, I'll teach some of the options you may have in the most common "hot spots."

It also helps to know who performs these attacks. Although muggers tend to be from disadvantaged environments, rapists are from no particular ethnic group or income level. Despite street talk and stereotypical clichés that suggest otherwise, whites usually rape whites, Hispanics most times rape Hispanics, blacks typically rape blacks. If someone is going to rape you, you'll most likely be attacked *not* by a stranger, by some "bad guy" you've never seen before and will never encounter again; over seventy-five percent of sexual assaults occur at the hands of someone you know, a person with whom you've developed a level of trust. The percentage of these crimes that go unreported is higher than any other. Many attacks of this sort happen because the person being assaulted did not react quickly. This is not her fault. The attacker uses his victim's trust to his advantage.

The best first line of defense, whether with an acquaintance or a stranger, is not necessarily to hit or kick 'em where it counts, but simply to be aware. Very many sexual attacks happen on dates. Before you decide to date a man for the first time, become aware of his general attitude toward women. Does he spout clichés about women? Does he view women as sexual objects? Does he tell jokes or make derogatory comments about women? Does he speak in general terms about women instead of seeing people as individuals? How interested is he in you as a person? Does he seem to view you as a conquest? Trust your instincts. If you don't like the answers you receive to these questions, you probably don't need to go out with this guy.

Even when you feel comfortable with a man, on early dates you may find it best to have another couple along and/or go with him only to public places. It's a good idea to carry a few quarters with you so you can make phone calls should you wish or need to. Among the most important questions you should ask yourself on these dates are: Does he encourage or allow me to have opinions that differ with his own? Does he seem uncomfortable with decisions I make for myself or for him? Does he patronize or speak "down" to me? Does he push drugs or alcohol on me when I don't want them?

In addition to the possibility of being raped by a fairly new acquaintance, you can be sexually assaulted by men with whom you've been intimate but with whom you no longer wish to have sex. Or you may be assaulted by someone you choose not to have sex with at a particular time. In the case of a former or current lover, it's important to recognize how well he respects your sexual limits.

It's no less possible, of course, that you'll be attacked by an absolute stranger. Your best protection, once again, is to have your antennae up. When you go out in public, as often as you can travel with a group of people. When you must go out alone, as you leave your house or building, pretend you're getting ready to cross the street. Always look both ways before, and as, you step. Watch those people around you; be aware of your surroundings at all times. Follow your instincts—if someone (or a group of people) looks like trouble, don't take the chance. Cross with seeming confidence to the other side of the street. Near dusk and at night, be conscious of shadows and avoid them. If one side of a street is better lighted than the other, take the lighted side. Swing wide around corners instead of walking close to walls—if someone plans to jump you, this simple action can buy you a crucial moment or two of reaction time.

Don't make yourself a target. It's not wise to look wealthy: Leave expensive jewelry at home when you go out unaccompanied. Conspicuous materialism may encourage a mugging. When you go out alone, try to wear clothing that allows a full range of movement should you need to respond to an attack. Jeans or slacks and a non-restrictive shirt are ideal. Perhaps the most important simple preventive action you can take, though, is to move always with purpose. Walk the walk of strength and confidence— take measured, self-contained steps, shoulders back, chest out, head level, awake and watchful, a little removed. Practice this walk (and look) at home in front of a full-length mirror. Predators are much less likely to feast on the woman who has a confident walk and powerful presence.

Should you choose to use any of the physical methods (strikes, kicks, etc.) in this book, there's no such thing as limited response. At the very least, attackers intend to seriously harm you. Muggings and beatings are obviously crimes of violence. So is rape. Date rape is rape. Sexual assault occurs every day without men penetrating their victims' bodies. If someone attempts to rape you or assault you in another way, these are violations not only of your body, but of your humanity. Muggings and beatings are no less violatory and are obviously just as dangerous as rape. Psychologists tell us that habitually violent criminals see their victims not as human beings but as *things* in their way—and sometimes as objects that can be used to satisfy one or another of their perceived needs. It goes without saying that someone who sees you as an object instead of as a person will probably have an easier time rationalizing torturing, maiming, or killing you. As women, we can't accept any justification for being treated as less than complete human beings.

A 120-pound woman being assaulted by a 190-pound man is at a major disadvantage. The attacker is far stronger, more powerful, and is genetically predisposed to be a whole lot more aggressive than you. If you're like most women, you've had little experience as a fighter. Many men, on the other hand, have had a considerable number of actual fights. This gives your attacker a huge environmental advantage. You must train to offset your liability. Most of the techniques in this book are simple; all of the techniques in this book are practical. They can be used with grand effectiveness by most people. There's minimal likelihood of success, however, if you put this manual in a drawer and do not refer to it. You must regularly practice. Planning, practice, and energized commitment are the keys to not freezing when you're attacked. Set aside a minimum of fifteen minutes each day to plan and practice. Find partners to practice with, preferably males (someone you like: maybe your mate or brother) who aren't afraid to be aggressive with you. It's best to work with several partners, of different sizes, styles of movement, levels of strength, speed, and aggressiveness. The best place to find these people could be in a martial arts school. Unfortunately, however, there are very few martial arts schools that provide the kind of reality training that you need. Near the end of the book, I've included a few tips about how to find a good school.

It's also helpful on a regular basis to practice the techniques alone. Practice when you get up in the morning, on your way to the shower, while preparing meals, and while watching TV. Practice saying "no!" forcibly and repeatedly. When you say "no!" it can't sound tentative or wimpy; it must sound as if it's a commandment straight from God. Practice yelling with authority. This sort of yelling can have a similar effect to the walk of strength: It can be a deterrent. The correct yell is one of confidence, strength, assertiveness. In addition to startling an attacker, yelling can empower you; it's a release, it wakes you up (helps you realize when you're attacked or in trouble that this is no movie you're watching—this is real life), and prepares you to do that which is necessary. It also might alert others in the vicinity that you're in trouble.

Imaging is another extremely beneficial technique. Imagine what you'll do when you're attacked in different situations. Learn to think like a warrior. Plan and practice at every opportunity. Practice always with an almost crazed level of intensity. Practice until these techniques become part of you. If you don't practice regularly and in a way that attempts to replicate reality, when you are attacked you'll most likely fail.

If you're going to fight, it's usually best to *fight early*, to fight before your attacker gets momentum going. Fight before he shoves you in your car. Fight before he picks you up and carries you down the alley. Fight before he throws you up against the wall. Fight before he restrains your arms and/or legs. Fight before, while sitting on your sofa, he punches you and tells you to bend over. Fight before your attacker knows you intend to fight. And fight with absolute commitment.

Lots of women are understandably squeamish about the idea of gouging out a man's eyes, crushing his genitals and esophagus, breaking his knees and elbows. When attacked, you can't afford to hesitate or to hold anything back. If, in the hopes of discouraging an attacker, you attempt to stick your fingers into his eyes just a little bit, there's an extreme likelihood that this will not be enough to discourage him. Indeed, you may incite even more violent acts; he may kill you. Some attackers enjoy the fight; some like pain being inflicted upon them. To survive, you must strike the weakest points on your assailant(s). And you must do so with no morals, without hesitation, with your most powerful available weaponry—whether this means fingers, knees, teeth, ballpoint pen, or a canister of pepper spray—and with absolute intention of dramatically damaging him (them). For example, in more than fifty percent of all rapes performed by one assailant, fellatio is forced with no weapon in evidence: *Use your teeth in the most effective ways you can.* Men are extremely vulnerable at the moment of orgasm; when a rapist "comes," you may choose to bite his penis as hard as you can. You may even find a similarly opportune moment long before he has an orgasm. This attitude will give you your best chance for survival. When attacked, survival is triumph enough.

OTHER IMPORTANT POINTS TO REMEMBER

You're never in a position to walk away clean from an attack.

If you've suffered physical injury, the first step should be to go to a hospital or to your personal doctor. This is no less true even if you don't believe you've been physically harmed; it's vital to be sure you've not sustained internal injuries. In addition, in the case of rape, you'll probably be more comfortable finding out if you're pregnant, and you'll want to receive testing for sexually transmitted diseases.

While at the hospital or doctor's office, I suggest you call a crisis hotline to ask what to do next. A qualified and empathetic counselor can be of enormous help. If you've not been physically hurt, you'll still have considerable emotional trauma to deal with. Rape counselors tell us that almost every victim feels misplaced guilt. "I could've, should've (or shouldn't have) done this, that, or the other," victims think. This is called survivor's guilt. Crisis hotlines can help you find proper counseling. The sooner you get counseling, the better the recovery goes. Crisis hotlines can also help you decide if you want to report the crime. It will be important for you to empower yourself, to make your own decision as to whether or not you want to file a report.

It's probably fair to suggest that many local legal systems are less than enlightened. Traditionally, society has blamed the victim for being attacked: "What did you do to encourage the attacker?" has been a typical response. As women, we must recognize that, just as there's no reason to feel guilt over having been assaulted, we need not feel guilty over defending ourselves in the most effective ways we can learn. Should we choose not to defend ourselves, this choice is no reason for guilt either. There's no rule that says you have to fight or that you even should fight. When attacked, if you choose to fight, you may find that this behavior doesn't work; your instincts may tell you it's best to stop being assertive. (There is hardly a way to overstate the value of listening to your instincts in this as well as many other situations that I'll describe in the book.) There are times when submission may be the ploy to get through an attack alive. Anything may be the ploy. Survival is the goal. Do whatever it takes to survive.

As you practice the skills in this book, decide what you can realistically do. Ask yourself if you believe you'll be emotionally capable of putting out an attacker's eyes. If after considerable physical practice and imaging you decide that you can't, it might be best to support yourself with an effective form of weaponry other than your hands and feet (see Simple Weaponry on page 109).

It's also wise to know the legal responsibilities of your decision to defend yourself. Some courts of law may consider defensive actions described in this book to be excessive. As society becomes more enlightened as to the nature of physical assaults against women, perhaps it will be more common for people to understand that we must do whatever is necessary to defend ourselves.

Basic Fitness Training for Survival

When performing a physical task, the more fit you are, the better you'll execute. While it's not necessary to be a world-class athlete to defend yourself, the person who is fit has a better chance not only to escape but to inflict damage with strikes. In addition, someone who is fit and feels good about herself has a more confident walk, a powerful presence that can help keep attackers at a distance, and is more likely to be awake to her surroundings. Perhaps most importantly, it gives her the ability to conquer self-doubt and to empower herself.

I want to stress that many of the following seemingly standard calisthenic and aerobic exercises have been altered from their traditional forms. The purpose is to use these exercises and drills to develop self-defense skills, not simply for their more standard benefits.

CARDIOVASCULAR TRAINING

Running

It's important never to run within an hour after having eaten a meal. When running, light porous clothing should be worn. In winter months, insulate yourself against the elements. You should wear a hood and/or a knit cap to protect the ears, and gloves or mittens to avoid damage that can easily be done to hands in cold weather.

Before beginning your run, perform a few minutes of stretching exercises.

It's best to run on resilient terrain, so as not to suffer damage to the hips, groin, and legs. When running, breathe in and out through the nose, not the mouth. Run on the balls of your feet; this will condition your legs to be more mobile when fighting. Imagine an assailant in front of you, at whom you *must* launch attacks and counters. As you become well conditioned, work toward sprinting the last several hundred yards of your run. As you complete the run, cool down by walking at least five minutes. To lessen muscle soreness, massage muscle groups.

Jumping Rope

You may wish to jump rope instead of, or in addition to, running. Rope jumping is among the best of aerobic exercises. It develops balance, relaxation, synchronization of hand and foot movement, timing, speed, and agility—all qualities that are helpful should you need to defend yourself.

As children, almost all of us skipped rope. Few of us did it properly.

The best jump rope is leather or plastic cord. The length of the rope depends on your height, but most women are able to use an eight-foot rope. Jump ropes are not expensive pieces of equipment. You can probably buy a good one for less than ten dollars. Until you buy a rope, you can substitute a section of plastic clothesline or a cloth rope. If a cloth rope is used, to give a little extra weight to the rope and thereby make it turn faster, duct tape can be wrapped around a two-foot section near the middle of the rope.

The correct way to begin jumping rope is to stand with your back and legs straight and your feet together. Look straight ahead. Place the rope at the heels of your feet and in a relaxed manner hold the handles of the rope slightly away from the sides of your body. In one motion, swing the rope up behind your back, over your head, and down across your body. As the rope nears your feet, with straight legs, make a small jumping motion (one to two inches off of the floor). Be sure to stay on the balls of your feet when jumping.

This is the basic rope jumping technique from which all variations flow. It's tougher than it sounds. Don't become discouraged when you can't immediately do it. The most common mistakes beginners make are to bend their knees when jumping and to try too hard. Beginners almost always become winded pretty quickly. Relax. It'll take practice to master the basic technique.

As you become proficient, you'll find yourself wanting to try new movements with the rope. There are many rope techniques. Among the most common ones that don't take long to master are jumping one foot at a time; jumping one foot in front of the other; jumping toe first, then heel first; and raising one leg to a ten count, then the other (a terrific balance builder).

A training tip:

When working with the rope, think about *gaining* energy by jumping, not about losing it.

SECONDARY AEROBIC EXERCISES

Aerobics classes, tennis, handball, dancing, bicycling, basketball, cross-country skiing, and table tennis are all stamina-building activities that can be performed instead of, or in addition to, running or jumping rope. Many of these activities develop attributes such as rhythm, hand-eye coordination, and timing, that can help should you find yourself in a situation where you choose to defend yourself.

ARM, CHEST, BACK, AND SHOULDER EXERCISES

The triceps, chest, back, and shoulders are the most important muscle groups for hand strikes. Bicep and shoulder muscles are the lifting and throwing muscle groups. The sort of bulkiness that is created by regularly pushing heavy weights, and is encouraged in most weight-lifting gyms, is not conducive to self-defense. The most efficient body, the one that allows a full range of motion, is lithe. Calisthenics help develop this body type more than any other form of exercise.

Push-ups

Many women can't do a full (men's) push-up. The correct women's push-up is performed on your knees, with your head raised, looking straight ahead at all times. Hands should be pointed forward. Your chin and chest should brush the floor when lowering your body. Push-ups should be done every day. Start by doing one set until the point of failure. After one week, increase to two sets. When you can do three sets of twenty-five with only one minute's rest between sets, try to do a few full (men's) push-ups.

The correct full push-up is performed with your

body in one line, buttocks tucked—not protruding. Everything else about the basic form is much the same as the women's push-up. Full push-ups will probably be very difficult at first. Don't become discouraged. Work hard. You'll feel your strength level grow as you work. And you'll find you become a more effective manager of your body, which is of enormous benefit when practicing personal defense techniques and, of course, when you find it necessary to use them.

Other upper body exercises

Muscle groups of the chest, shoulders, and back are strengthened by working out on a rowing machine, by doing pull-ups (inexpensive door-mount bars are sold in most sporting goods stores), and by "walking" across a ladder that has been mounted horizontally. The ladder is a particularly useful piece of equipment that, in addition to strengthening the desired muscle groups, develops agility and teaches you to coordinate movement of the left side of your body with the right. Ladders of this kind can be found on most children's playgrounds and in many gyms.

HAND AND FOREARM EXERCISES

Considerable power in short hand strikes can be gained from developing strong forearms. Strong hands enable you to move an attacker into position to receive blows.

Common handgrips work well to serve these ends, as does a small handball, which can be held in the palm of your hand and tightly squeezed, without using your thumb. An excellent invention is the soft Styrofoam keychain that is molded to fit your hand. These are sold by many martial arts training equipment companies. Another useful device is a common newspaper. Sheets of newsprint can be tightly curled in your palm, again without using your thumb. I suggest you perform several hundred repetitions with any of these every day.

LEG EXERCISES

Most people are surprised to learn that much of the power in hand techniques is generated from the legs. The major power groups in your legs are the front thigh (quadriceps) and calf muscles. The following exercises will help develop these muscle groups.

Knee bends

Knee bends help establish proper balance as well as build necessary power in the legs. The correct knee bend is done with your back straight and your legs spread fairly wide. Bend straight down until the backs of your thighs touch the underside of your calves. Be sure to keep both feet flat on the floor.

Perform a minimum of twenty-five repetitions every other day.

Squat thrusts

On a count of one, drop to a squatting position with legs spread and hands between your legs. On a count of two, shoot your legs out behind your body in a push-up like position. On three, tuck your legs back into a squatting position. On four, jump as high as possible and reach for the ceiling. Begin with twelve repetitions every other day. Over a period of weeks, increase to fifty reps.

Important:

Be sure to jump high at the end of every rep. This helps you create mobility and power in your legs.

Calf raises

Stand straight, with your feet six to eight inches apart. Raise the heel of both feet from the floor as high as you comfortably can. Hold for a two count, then lower to a four count. Perform a minimum of fifty repetitions every other day.

ABDOMINAL EXERCISES

Sit-ups

The basic sit-up is performed on the floor, with your hands behind your head and with legs spread and knees bent. Try to do at least fifteen repetitions per day, at least five days a week. You should soon move up to twenty-five repetitions per set, then fifty.

Crunches

From the basic sit-up position, raise the upper body about six inches off of the floor and hold for a one to two second count at the top of the motion. Perform as many repetitions as possible at least five days a week.

Initially, these will make your stomach muscles sore.

STRETCHING

I teach stretching not to make you a high kicker but because stretching will allow you to throw faster, more powerful kicks below waist height. Stretching also gives you a greater range of motion and reduces the likelihood of injury when you need to move quickly.

Stretching should be relaxed. Perform these movements slowly and easily. Simply exhale and gently lean into the stretch as far as you comfortably can, then continue to take deep, slow breaths as you hold the stretch. If your breathing becomes fast or strained, you're trying too hard.

Butterfly stretch

This exercise stretches the groin muscles and the muscles of the inner thigh.

The butterfly stretch is performed while sitting on the floor with your back erect, head facing straight ahead, with your legs spread yet bent at the knees, and the bottom of your feet pressed flat against one another. Place your elbows on your thighs slightly above each knee, grasping both ankles tightly. To execute the butterfly stretch, simply press down with both elbows on your thighs until maximum stretch is achieved—then hold this position to a count of twenty and release. It's important not to bounce your legs up and down when performing this, or any other, stretching exercise. The butterfly stretch should be repeated several times. Perform this exercise roughly five minutes every day.

Front stretch

Although this stretch primarily works the hamstrings, the groin muscles also come into play.

After finishing the butterfly stretch, remain seated on the floor and place your left leg straight out in front of your body. Next, bend your right leg at the knee and tuck the heel of your right foot in next to the right side of your buttocks. Spread both legs apart until they form an "L" shape.

Grasp the ball of your left foot with the palm of your left hand while placing the palm of your right hand on your left knee to keep that knee "locked" flat on the floor. Bend forward at the waist until you feel the stretch in the muscles just above the inside of your knee, then pull down slightly with your left hand and arm. When you feel that you can stretch no further, hold this position for a ten count. Take deep, slow breaths as you hold the stretch. Repeat this exercise five times with your left leg, then switch to your right.

As a beginner, you're likely to have a limited range of motion in these muscle groups, but with daily practice, you should eventually be able to place your nose on the floor to the inside of your knees.

Lower back and groin stretch

Sit with your back erect, legs spread to the sides in a comfortable position. Slowly lean forward from your hips, keeping your thigh muscles relaxed. Lean as far forward as possible and hold this position for thirty seconds. Stretch your hands to the front and place them on the floor for balance. With your knees locked, place the palm of your left hand around your left foot; pull forward and hold for a ten count; then do the same with your right leg. Repeat this stretch five times.

Basic Hand and Arm Strikes

Hand techniques are far and away the most versatile, effective, and practical weapons. Unlike kicks, hand techniques can be thrown with beautiful efficiency to the proper targets from almost any body position, with good stopping power, laser accuracy, blazing speed, and with quick recovery time between strikes.

Most of the hand techniques in this manual are open-handed strikes. It's usually best not to punch with a closed fist to the face. When you punch with a closed fist, you may be doing yourself a disservice and your attacker a favor. When fighting an attacker, the purpose is not to cause him a little discomfort by punching him on the nose, but to take him out as expeditiously as possible. It's very easy to damage your hands by throwing close-fisted punches. If you hurt your hand while poking someone on the jaw, you're probably not going to hit him again. By properly throwing open-handed strikes, there's far less risk of injuring your hands. Perhaps most importantly, there are many open-handed strikes that cause more severe punishment, and which are much more likely to incapacitate attackers than close-fisted punches.

It's imperative to use instantly debilitating techniques on the least protected targets. Primary targets for hand strikes, in order of importance, are:

1. eyes
2. throat
3. groin
4. elbows

Take note that if your attacker is wearing tight denim jeans, penetration for groin strikes with either the hands or the feet may be quite difficult. Groin strikes work well with nearly any other clothing.

Most of the simplest strikes are thrown linearly. In a majority of situations, a straight line strike is more effective than a strike that is thrown in an arcing or looping motion. This is true for several reasons: 1) it takes a looping strike longer to reach its target than a straight one, which 2) means the opponent is more likely to see it coming, thereby 3) being able to intercept it or even to time the blow and catch you throwing the strike with his own counterattack in the middle of your offensive movement, and 4) to loop a strike is to waste motion; the strike being thrown becomes less powerful and you become tired more quickly.

An Important Tip:

Many attackers will "telegraph" their intentions in one way or another. If you are alert, if you follow your instincts, and if you see a possible assailant from a distance, you may be able to spot something in the way he's watching you or in the manner that he approaches. This gives you the opportunity to act instead of react.

Untrained fighters usually launch inefficient punches, kicks, strikes, or they will attempt to grab you in a way that unintentionally lets you know that their attack has started. This gives you a very brief window of opportunity to strike your attacker before he can react. When you can strike someone before he has seen the attack and/or can react to it, the effect of your blows will be maximized.

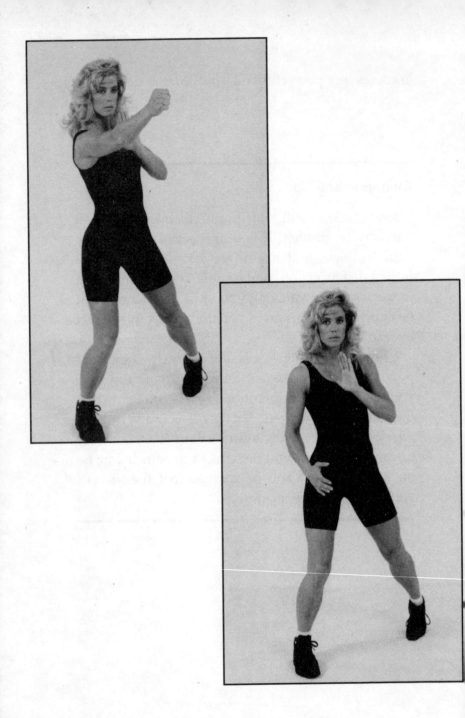

BASIC STRIKES

Lead-hand strike

The lead-hand strike will be the most versatile tool in your repertoire. It is the primary, first, and most important weapon. It is the strike upon which all others are based.

The lead-hand strike should be mastered before you learn to throw any other strikes. It is called the lead-hand strike because it is thrown, always, by the arm closest to the target. It is one of the fastest and most deceptive strikes; a proper lead-hand strike is thrown with explosive speed and quickness. It can often catch an attacker off guard. It is thrown with your hand closed in a fist and it travels straight away from your body.

Important: Please see photos below that show how to properly make a fist. Although this may seem trivial, it's not. Even professional boxers and kickboxers have broken their hands because they punched with an improperly made fist.

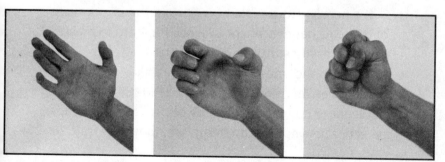

The lead-hand strike can be launched from many different positions—with hands all the way down at your sides, from a crossed-arms position (figure 1), and from the universal surrender position (figure 2), among others. Your hands and feet move synchronistically when throwing the strike. Penetration in the lead-hand strike comes from redistributing weight off of your rear leg and into your lead leg, and in angling your upper body toward the target. Your elbow should be locked at the moment of deepest impact and you should think not about simply reaching the target, but about driving the blow about a foot through. When facing your attacker, keep your eyes focused on the center of his chest throughout delivery of this and all blows.

One of the best ways to develop the lead-hand strike is by practicing it in front of a mirror. Throw a bare minimum of forty lead-hand strikes at your reflection in the mirror every day (this takes only a couple of minutes). Another way to work on this most basic of strikes is by throwing it at a sheet of notebook paper hung from the ceiling or in a doorway and suspended from a string.

It's nearly impossible to overstate the importance of the lead-hand strike or to work too hard to master this seemingly simplest of weapons.

Among the most common mistakes beginners make when learning to throw the lead-hand strike is not leaning far enough into the blow. This often happens because novices are tentative; they are afraid to

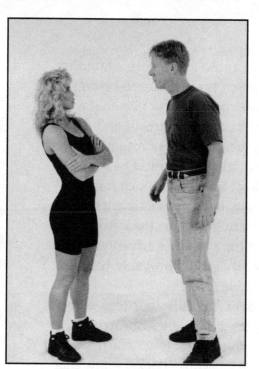

figure 1

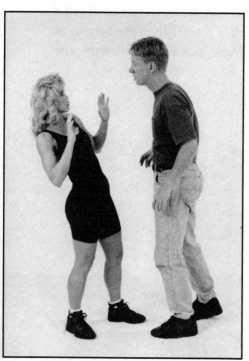

figure 2

commit themselves. I want to stress once again that your attacker is almost certainly going to be bigger and stronger and more experienced at personal warfare than you. You must commit yourself and do so totally. Remember that one advantage you may have is that of surprise. Your intention should be to shock your assailant by hitting him with as much force and as many times as you can to the most efficient targets before he knows you've initiated an attack. You can't afford to count on this (or any other advantage you believe you might have), but it's probable he'll not expect you to be a capable fighter.

Another common error is to lift your lead elbow up and away from your body when throwing the strike, thereby telegraphing the blow, which slows down delivery time and lets your attacker know that the strike is coming. To stand the best chance of your blow reaching its target, it's vital that the whole of your body works in a single line when throwing the lead-hand strike.

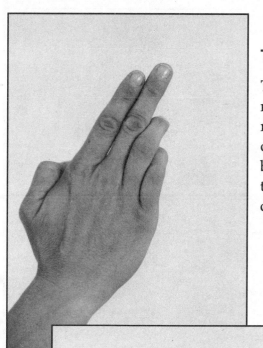

Two finger spear

Thrown with the index and middle fingers open and rigid, the last two fingers curled forward, the thumb back and out of the way, this technique is used exclusively to the eyes.

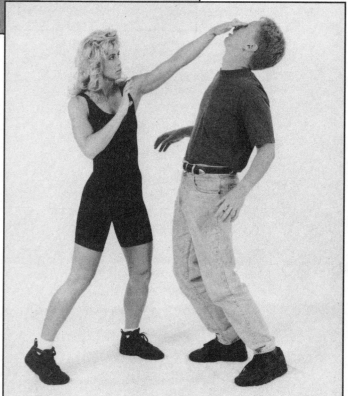

45

Straight claw/palm heel

The thumb is in the same position as with the two finger spear; all four fingers are open and rigid. Claw forcefully to the eyes and face and/or explosively shove the heel (bottom) of the palm to the nose or chin.

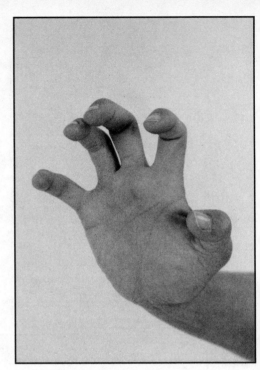

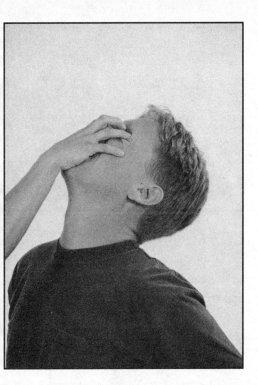

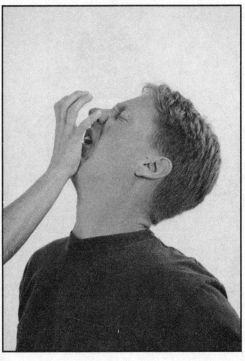

Open hand to the throat

The webbed space between the thumb and the index finger is open and is in a slightly cupped (arched) position (figure 1). Thrust with bad intentions deep into the Adam's Apple (figure 2).

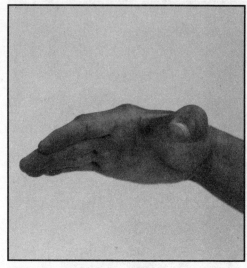

figure 1

figure 2

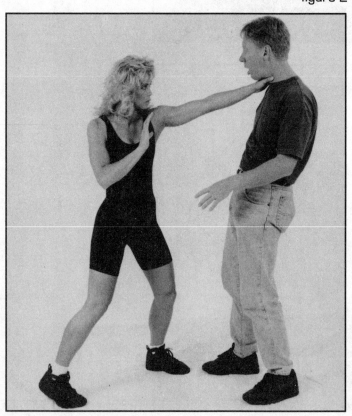

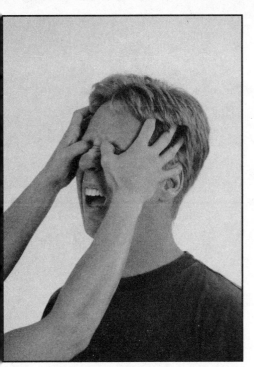

Thumb gouge

The hand is held in the same positioning as the open hand to the throat strike. This technique is often thrown simultaneously with both hands. Plunge deeply into the eyes (figure 3).

figure 3

Groin grabs

Groin grabs are performed when you're attacked from either the front (figure 1) or the rear (figure 2). Your fingers are held open and are fairly relaxed. Quickly grab the testicles (figure 3). Squeeze as hard as you can.

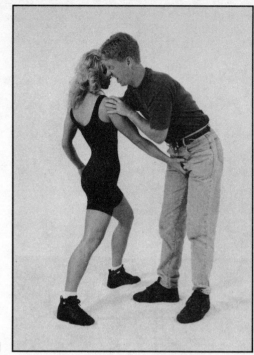

figure 1

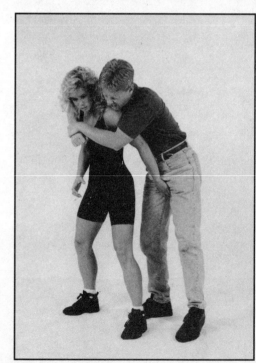

figure 2

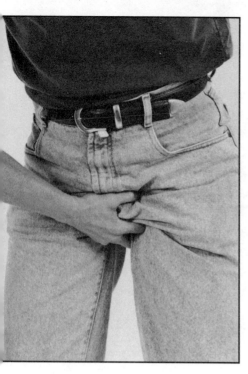

figure 3

Important:

This is a straight line technique. Do not waste motion. Throw it as cleanly as possible. Do not grab the penis. This will cause the assailant little damage (other than fright); be sure to reach under the groin for the testicles.

Hammer fist

This closed-fist technique is typically thrown at an angle similar to that of a hammer making contact with a nail.

Contact is made with the fleshy outside of your hand. The hammer fist is a concussively powerful blow that is thrown to the base of the skull and, when you have locked an attacker's arm, to the elbow. Compared to most strikes, the hammer fist has a slow delivery time. It's best not to try to use it as a lead technique; you're most likely to use the hammer fist as a follow-up blow.

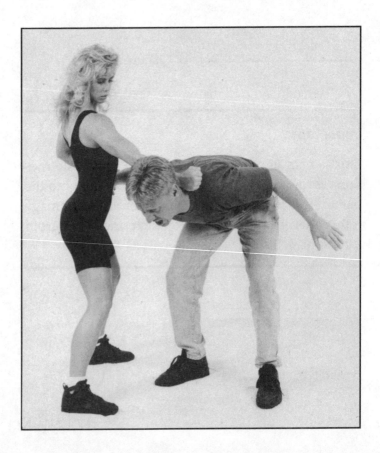

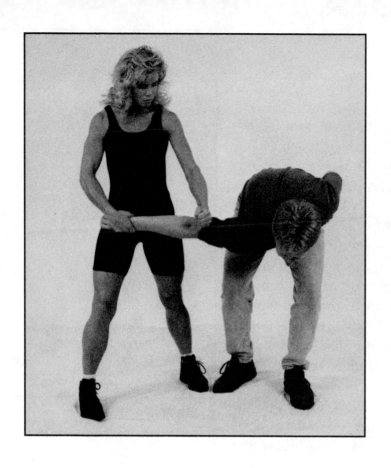

Hammer backfist

This strike, which will most often be used as a follow-up blow, has the same hand configuration as the hammer fist. Like the basic lead-hand strike, the hammer backfist is always thrown from the side closest to your attacker. Unlike the hammer fist, it can be launched from numerous hand and arm positions. Like the lead-hand strike, the hammer backfist takes regular practice to master.

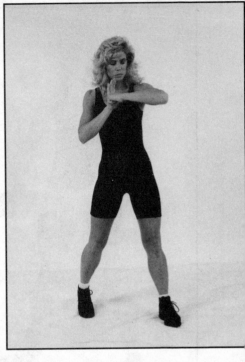

To learn to throw the hammer backfist, bend your arm at the elbow and tuck it in close to your body. Snap the lower half of your arm out from your body in an explosive, whipping action. As is true of the basic lead-hand strike, a properly executed hammer backfist has a similar velocity to a boxer's jab.

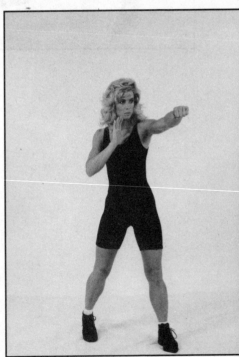

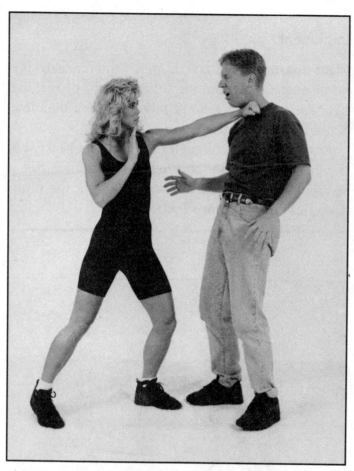

The primary target for the hammer backfist is the Adam's Apple.

Important:

Many martial arts students make the (conceivably fatal) mistake of "pulling" this punch, of making light surface contact; don't forget to drive the blow about a foot through the target.

Another primary target for the hammer backfist is the groin. A hammer backfist to the groin is not a snapping punch; concentrate on digging the blow deep into the assailant's body.

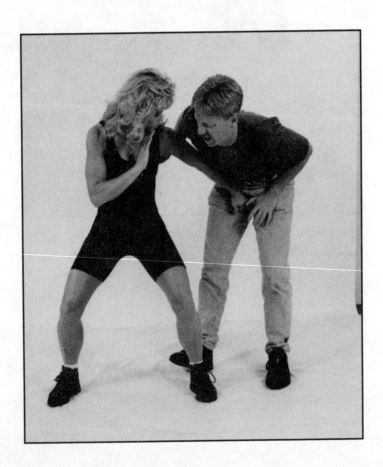

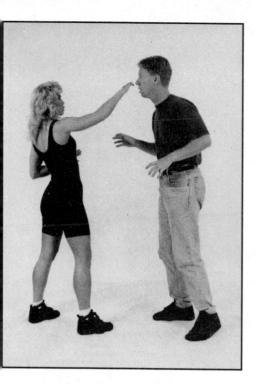

Raking claw

The raking claw is used exclusively to the eyes and is thrown from almost identical angles as those of the hammer backfist to the throat. The differences are that this is an open-handed strike that is used in a flicking manner, with emphasis on accuracy instead of power, and that it will usually be a first strike. The tips of your fingers are dragged across the assailant's eyes.

If it connects properly, it can immediately, although temporarily, blind your attacker. With practice, many people can throw the raking claw with mercurial quickness. It's best not to think of the raking claw as a finishing blow, but one that will set up your attacker for his demise.

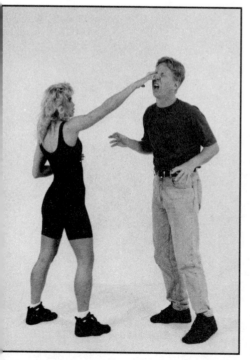

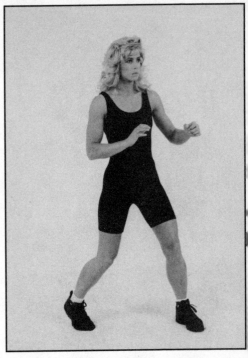

figure 1

Roundhouse elbows

Roundhouse elbows are thrown from both the lead and rear arms. The lead roundhouse elbow is thrown by rotating your lead shoulder (figure 1) and moving that elbow and arm explosively across the center of your chest (figure 2), at the same time pivoting your lead foot in an identical motion to the strike being thrown (figure 3).

The power in a rear roundhouse elbow springs from the legs and from a properly synchronized pivoting motion of the upper and lower body when delivering the blow. Your legs should be slightly bent at the knees. As you launch the rear roundhouse elbow, pivot on the ball of your rear foot at precisely the same angle and time as the strike being thrown, shifting your weight from your

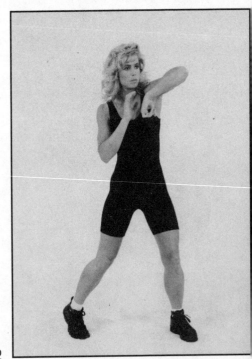

58

figure 2

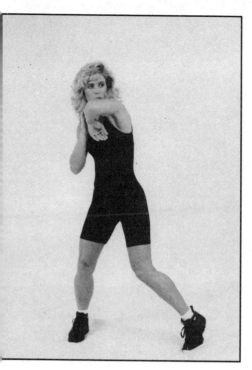

figure 3

rear leg to your front (figure 4).

These techniques sound much more difficult than they are in practice. Novices often make the mistake of cocking the arm before launching roundhouse elbows, thereby telegraphing the blows. Regular practice in front of a mirror is the best way to correct errors and to perfect the mechanics of this and all other strikes.

As always, it's important to focus your eyes on the assailant's chest throughout the trajectory of the strike. This tends to concentrate the power of the blow.

The most effective roundhouse elbows to the head land on the lower, center side of the jaw or to the temple.

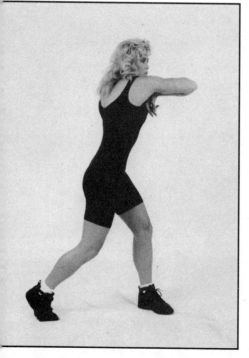

figure 4

Basic Foot and Leg Strikes

In many cases, more power can be generated with the legs than with the arms. Most women's legs are much stronger than their arms and are fairly equal in strength to men's. It should be stressed, however, that this does not make kicks nearly as effective as hand strikes.

No matter what's taught in your neighborhood karate class, there are few times when you should kick above groin level. Primary targets for kicks include:

1. knees
2. groin

There are several secondary targets for kicking techniques. Secondary targets are used as distractions and irritants; although they're not the core of your intent, they distract the assailant and open holes to drop in the heavy artillery. Secondary targets include:

1. insteps
2. shins
3. quadriceps
4. inside of the thighs

Note:

Other secondary targets are mentioned in the following descriptions of kicks and leg strikes.

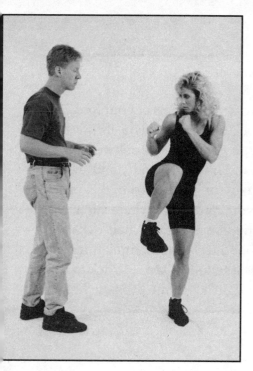

BASIC STRIKES

Sidekick

Although this kick is taught in almost every karate school in the world, its most practical applications are often neglected. For effective stopping power, there's seldom a reason to throw the sidekick to any target other than the knee. It's a very difficult kick to defend against when it's thrown in the following manner: chamber your leg—draw it in close to your body, folding it at the knee—then explode from this tucked position with bone-shattering commitment.

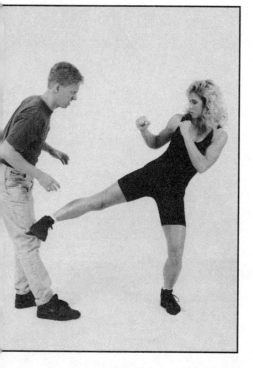

Important:

Be sure to make contact with the heel of your foot. Do not look at your attacker's knee as you throw the kick: This will telegraph your intent. Look instead at the center of his chest. His entire body, and every movement he can make, can be read from this position. With practice, you can know where his knee will be without looking directly at it. When kicks are thrown, as is true of hand techniques, think through the target. It's often best to follow the sidekick to the knee with a hard hand strike to the eyes or throat.

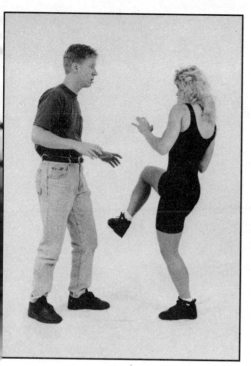

Oblique kick

This is a stomping technique that is thrown with your rear foot at a forty-five-degree outward angle. The intent is to stomp the attacker's knee with the heel of your foot. The beauty of this technique is that no chamber is required; it is, therefore, nearly nontelegraphic—in other words, it's very difficult for your assailant to see it coming. Again, do not look at the target; watch the center of his chest.

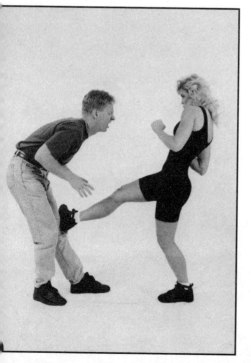

figure 1

Front kick

Front kicks are thrown with both the lead and rear foot. Pull your knee in close to your body, pointing it toward your intended target (figure 1), then shove your leg explosively away from your body. Front kicks are thrown with the ball of your foot to the groin (figure 2), to the knee (figure 3), thigh, bladder, and solar plexus. When you throw it to these targets, it's to be executed with both snap and thump. As always, think through the target. It's also thrown with the instep (or better yet, with the shin) to the groin (figure 4). When using a front kick to the groin, target deep; think about placekicking a football; lift your leg explosively into the testicles. A rising shin to the groin is amazingly effective from behind, and only slightly less marvelous

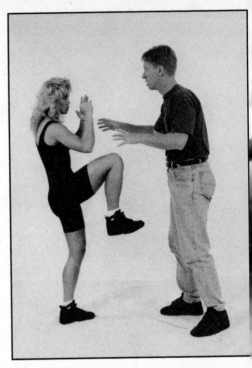

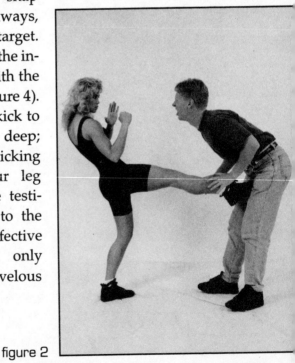

figure 2

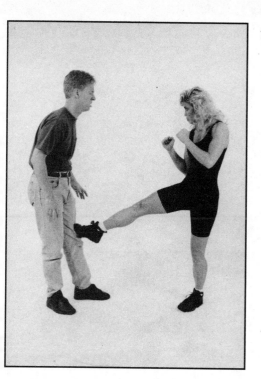

figure 3

from the front. It's often useful to follow the front kick with a well-placed, intensely committed hand strike to the eyes or throat.

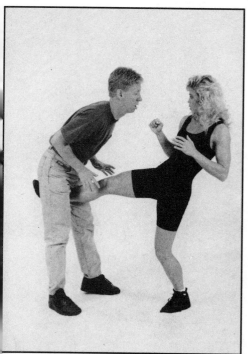

figure 4

67

Heel stomp

Lift your lead knee, then stomp with murderous intent with your heel.

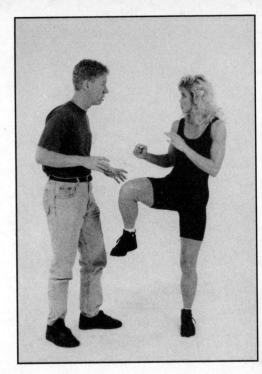

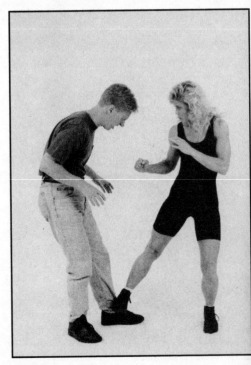

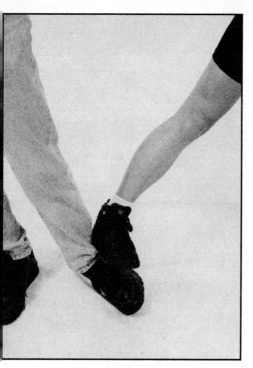

Targets:

If the attacker is standing, stomp his instep or ankle; if he's prone, stomp the groin, the throat, the temple.

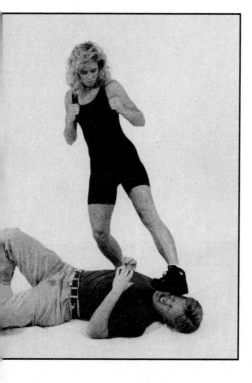

Striking Combinations

Odds are that you'll not be able to take out an attacker with one or two strikes. It is, therefore, imperative that you learn to throw arm and leg strikes in crisp, elegantly efficient combinations. Good combinations flow from natural, synchronized movement of the body. When practicing combinations, use all four of your basic tools—your lead and rear arms and legs—and begin as well as finish with your lead arm.

Perfect all strikes and combinations so that proper weapons are available to use against any conceivable attacker. No one needs to be at a disadvantage because she didn't learn to use a particular strike or combination of strikes to the best available target(s).

When throwing combinations that include kicks and/or leg strikes, it's often best to begin with a hand technique (figure 1), then a leg technique (figures 2 and 3), and finish with a hand strike (figure 4). Combinations of this design are more deceptive and balanced (translation: much more effective), and are more likely to finish the job.

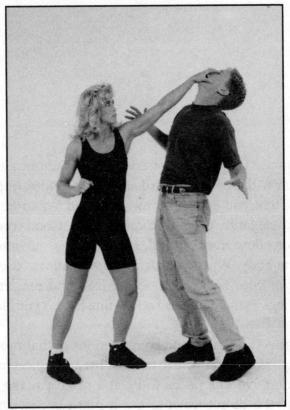

figure 1

Be inventive. When practicing, create your own simple, clean, efficient combinations of basic strikes.

It's seldom wise or efficient to attempt to kick your attacker above his waist. High kicks are often dangerous not for the person being kicked, but for the

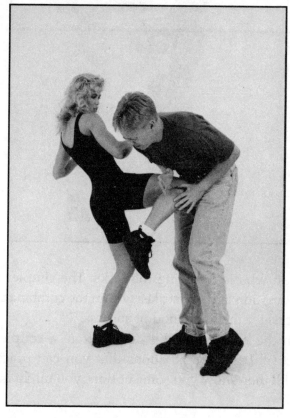

figure 2

(continued)

figure 3

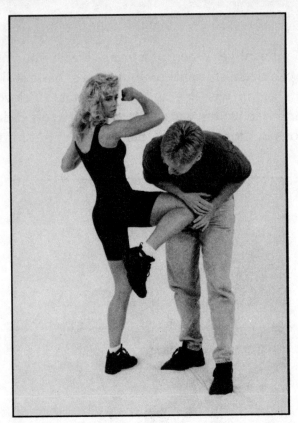

person who is throwing the kicks. The simpler the combination and the strikes within the combination, the greater the likelihood of success.

On the next pages, I'll demonstrate a couple of effective, basic combinations that you can practice and I'll then show you some options you might have

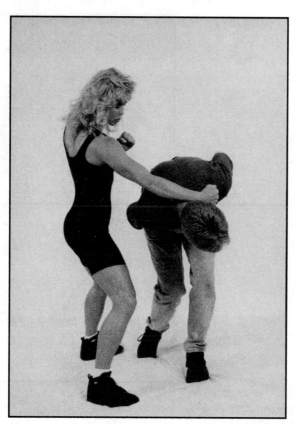

figure 4

in actual self-defense situations. You need to recognize, however, that in combat, combinations are usually fairly instinctive—they flow from the natural actions and reactions of your attacker, not from set routines.

An aggressor reaches for you.

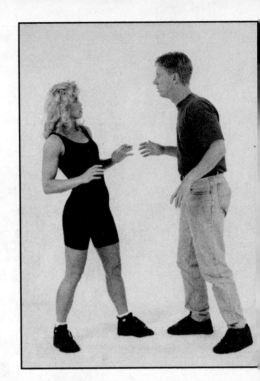

You short-circuit his attack by thrusting an open hand straight into his windpipe.

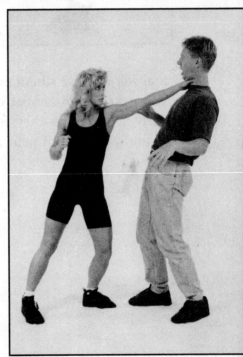

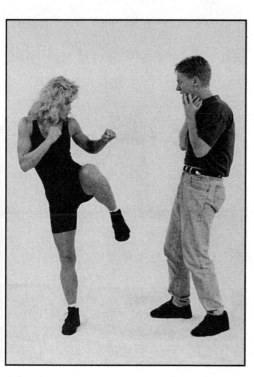

Quickly chamber your leg.

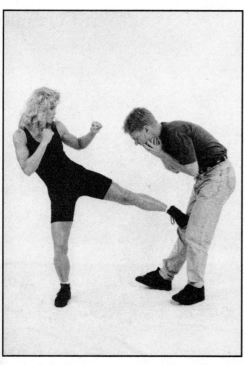

As he bends forward, reacting to your strike to his throat, use your lead leg to sidekick the front of his knee.

(continued)

NO! NO! NO!   77

Grab him forcefully by the
hair with both hands.

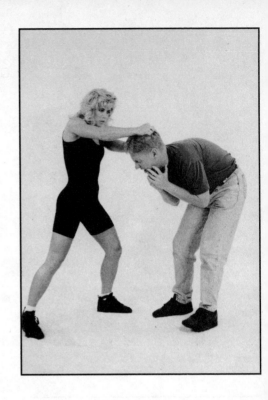

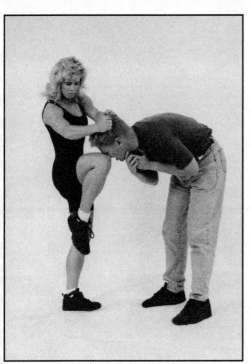

With your rear leg, knee him as hard as you can flat on the face. Immediately leave the attack site.

An attacker reaches for your front shoulder.

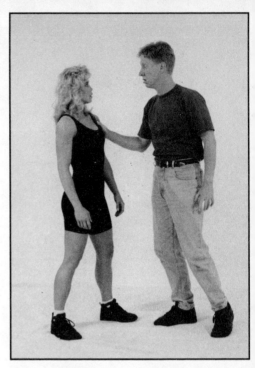

With your lead hand, instantly rake him across the eyes.

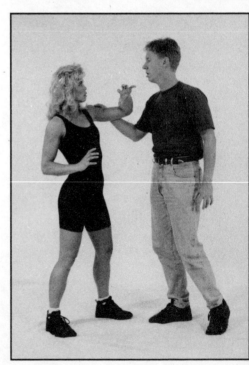

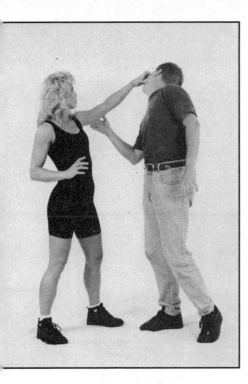

As he reacts to your strike by covering his face . . .

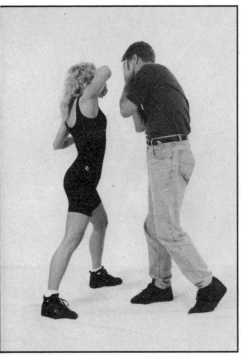

. . . launch a roundhouse elbow with your rear arm,
which slams into his temple.

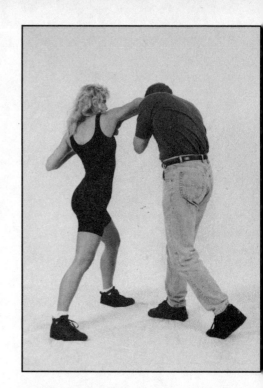

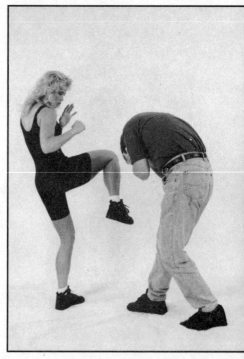

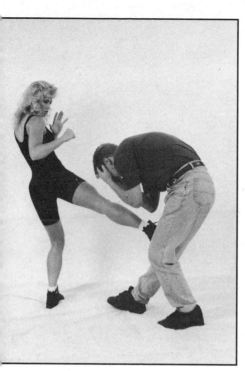

Finish him with a sidekick to his knee, and quickly leave the place of the attack.

"Real-life" Scenarios

As I mentioned in the introduction, it can help to know where you'll most likely be attacked. The vast majority of all violence against women takes place not on subways, in parking lots, alleys, or public rest rooms, but in victims' homes. In your house or apartment, as anywhere, prevention is the best line of defense. A few simple security rules and a bit of mind-set readjustment can go a long way.

First off, be careful; don't assume that just because you're at home, everything is okay. When there's a knock or the doorbell rings, don't blindly answer the door. If you don't have peepholes in your doors, install them. Always lock your doors and windows when you go out, even if only for a moment. When you return home, if something doesn't seem right, don't go in. If there are indications that someone may have broken into your house (lights that you left on are off; there's a draft in the middle of winter when you believe you had closed all of the windows; you see broken glass), don't enter. People feel violated when their possessions are taken from their homes. They often react as if in shock. If you unlock your door and see that your stereo and/or your TV is missing, don't go in. With antennae up and radar on, go to a friend's place or to a pay phone and call the police.

Another typical hot spot for attacks is victims' vehicles. Roughly twenty-five percent of all rapes take place in victims' own cars. The typical pattern for these assaults, if they're performed by strangers, is this: You're walking to your car alone; you get shoved in as you open the door.

As always, very many of these assaults are avoidable just by taking the appropriate preventive action. Park your car in a well-lighted area visible to passersby. Always lock your car doors when you leave it (as well as when you're driving). Don't walk to your car alone unless you absolutely have to. Should you find it necessary to go to your car by yourself, carry a simple, nontelegraphic weapon, such as an open ballpoint pen (see Simple Weaponry). Carry your weapon in your strong hand and your keys in the other. Practice using your weak hand to lock and unlock your car doors. Don't try to carry weapon and keys in the same hand and don't put yourself in a position where you're standing at your car door, fumbling around in your purse or pockets to find your keys. Always watch on all sides as you approach your car. Get in your car as cautiously and expeditiously as possible.

Whether in your home, car or someplace else, when you're attacked, you'll probably be accosted from either the front or the rear, while you're standing, sitting, or lying down. The following are examples of techniques that can be applied to a large number of situations. I want to warn you, though, not to deceive yourself into thinking that this or any other set of "A, B, C" responses will work for you in the real world. There are literally billions of people who can attack you in billions of places at billions of moments. Each of these people and each of these situations will be different. Your response to an attack will be dictated not by these routines, but will be a reaction to the individual attacker in the particular environment at that exact moment.

DEFENSES AGAINST FRONTAL ATTACKS

1.) Attack in a Public Restroom

You are leaving a public restroom.

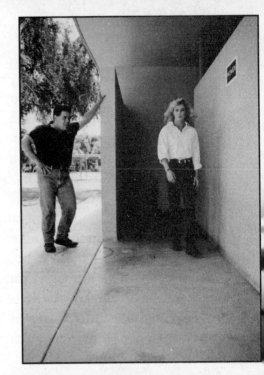

An awaiting attacker unexpectedly slams you into a wall, using both hands to grab you by the throat.

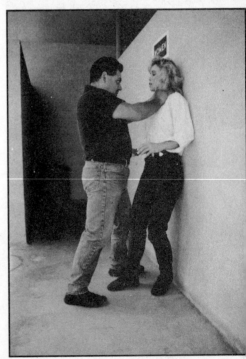

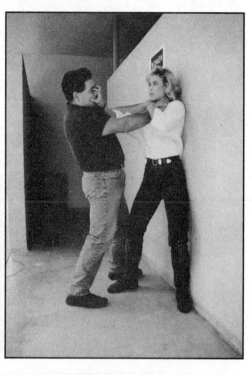

With your hands in a straight claw position, stick your fingers deeply into his eyes . . .

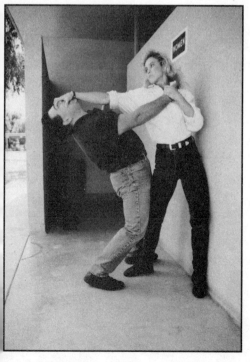

(*continued*)

NO! NO! NO!

. . . then push him off by his eyes, which gives you room to knee him in the testicles.

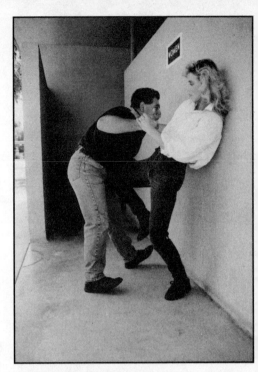

Hold his hand so he can't escape.

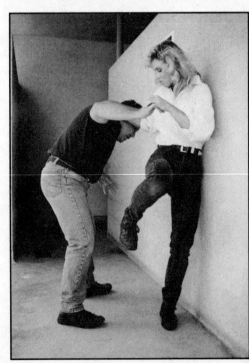

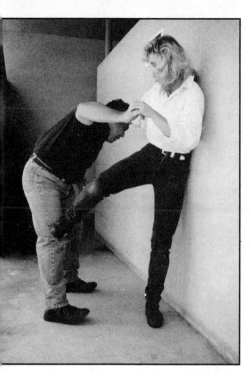

Break his knee with a side-kick, and leave the attack site.

2.) The "I Need Directions" Ploy

You are giving directions to a stranger.

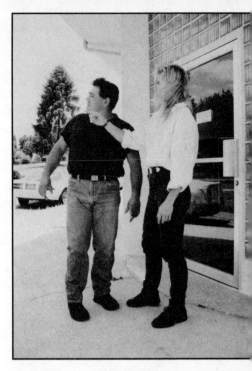

He surprises you by forcefully grabbing you with both hands around your waist.

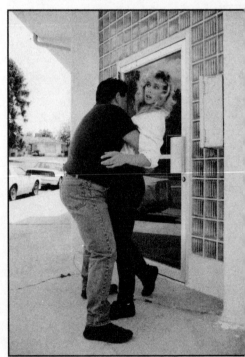

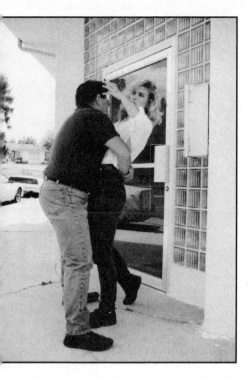

With your hands in the thumb gouge position, plunge both thumbs into his eyes.

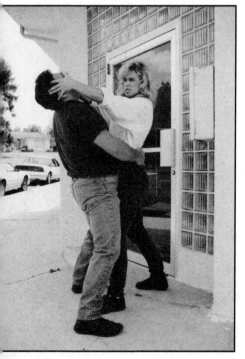

(*continued*)

Grab him forcefully by the hair.

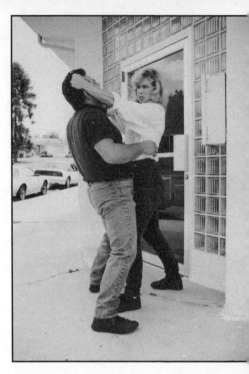

Pull his head down into your knee, and slam him in the face.

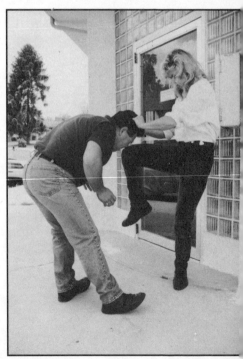

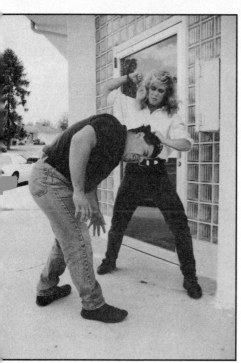

You hit him with a hammer-fist as hard as you can on the soft area at the base of his skull. As he falls, you make your escape.

DEFENSES AGAINST REAR ASSAULTS

1.) Surprise Attack from Behind

An attacker approaches from behind.

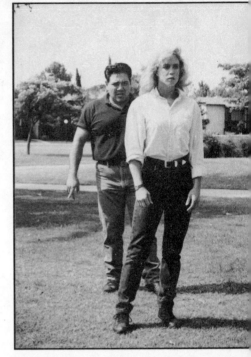

He grabs you with both hands in a choke hold.

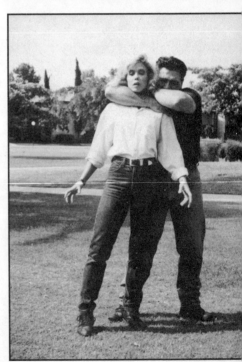

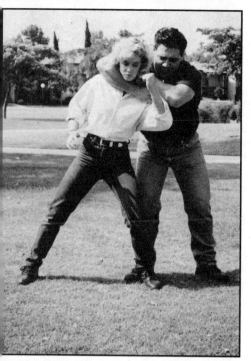

You gain balance and power positioning by stepping slightly to your right, where you raise your arm.

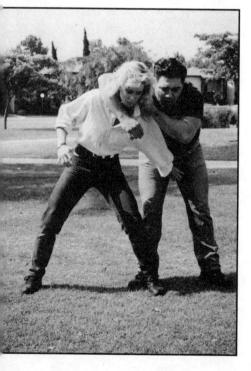

Drop your open hand to his testicles.

(continued)

Grab and squeeze as hard as you can.

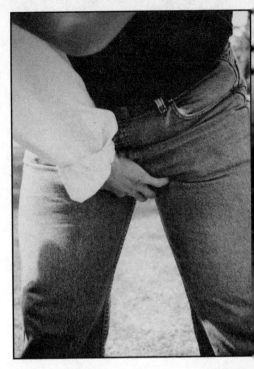

Let go and as he bends over, reacting to his pain, quickly chamber your leg.

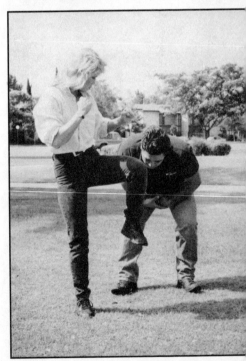

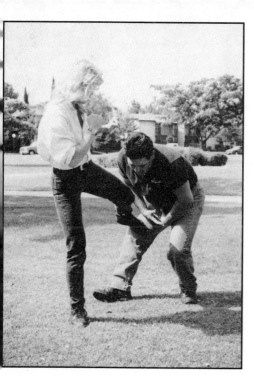

Snap a hard sidekick to his closest knee.

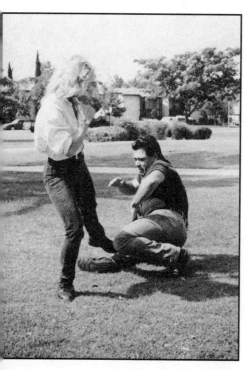

As he falls, leave.

2.) Surprise Attack from Behind

Your attacker approaches from behind.

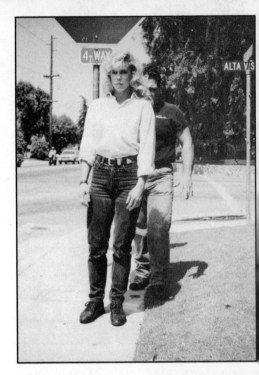

He grabs you by the shoulders.

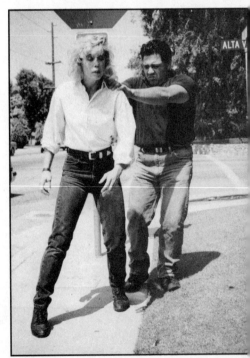

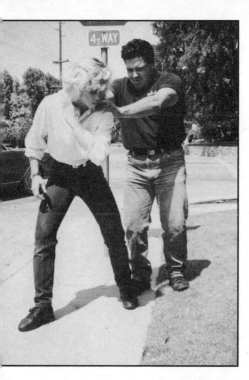

Step slightly to your right, raise your left hand and explosively snap it deep into your attacker's testicles.

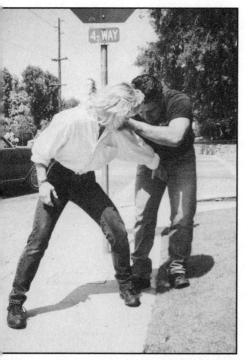

(continued)

As he reacts to his pain by bending forward, in a hitch-hike position, roll your thumb deeply into his eye. You then leave or, as necessary, finish him with an appropriate strike or strikes.

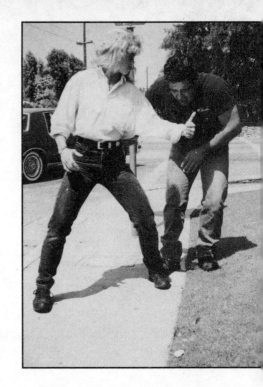

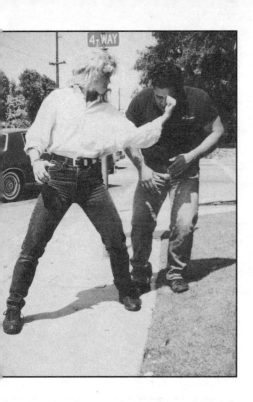

3.) "The Forced Kiss"

An attacker grabs you with both hands around your waist and leans toward you, to force a kiss.

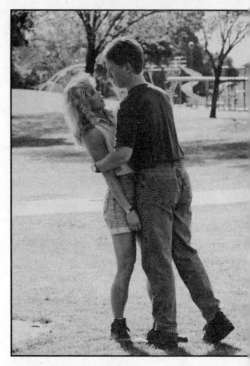

Bite his nose as hard as you can.

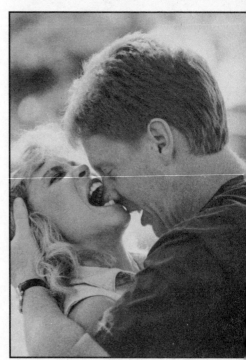

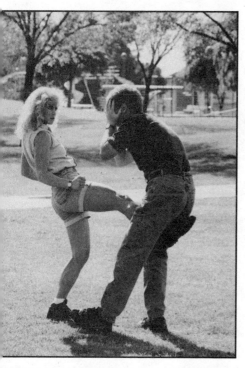

As he reaches for his nose and steps away in pain, use your shin to front kick him in the testicles. (Note: Think about lifting him a foot off of the ground.)

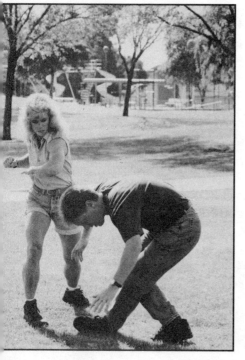

As he falls forward, you hasten his demise with a hard roundhouse elbow to the side of the head. Leave immediately.

DEFENSE AGAINST AN ATTACK IN A VEHICLE

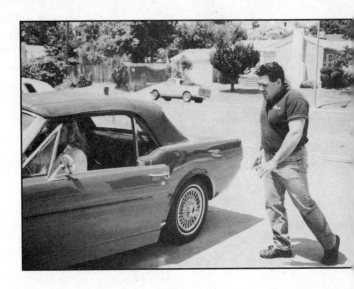

As you are getting out of or into your car, an attacker approaches. He places himself in the space between the door and the car.

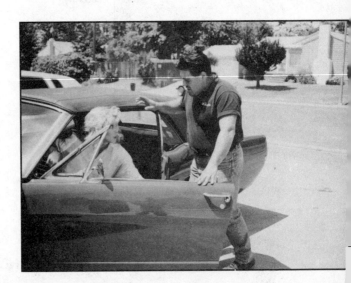

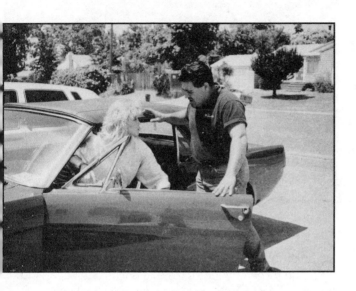

Step from your car. With your rear arm, claw him forcefully in the eyes (remember to think through the target).

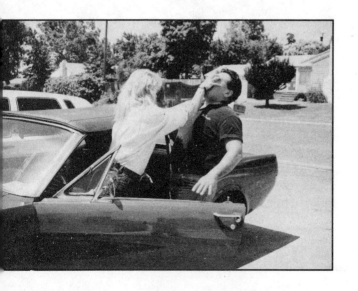

(*continued*)

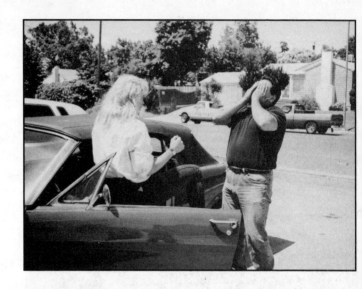

As he steps back and covers his eyes, reacting to the pain and force of your strike, dig a front kick deep into his groin. As he falls, get into your car and leave.

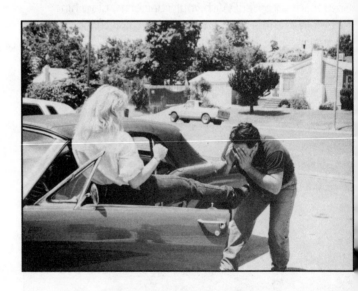

Simple Weaponry

Many martial arts schools and women's defense courses suggest car keys as the simple weapon of choice. Although this advice is of course well intentioned, it's dangerously wrong-minded and misinformed. It's almost impossible to use car keys with enough force to harm an attacker. Should you try to drive them into an assailant's eyes or throat, it's not only improbable that you'll be able to do so (thereby further angering someone who means to do you harm), you're also likely to hurt your hand in the attempt.

Perhaps the most efficient simple "non-weapon" form of weaponry is an open ballpoint pen tightly grasped in your writing hand (this is probably your strongest hand and the one that has the greatest dexterity) and reinforced with the thumb. A hammer backfist to an attacker's throat with this deceptively effective weapon is easily executed and conceivably lethal. If the throat isn't available or if you miss it, stab your attacker in any and every painful place you can: the cheeks, the hollow behind his ears, the neck, the arms, the stomach, the kidneys, the thighs. Puncture wounds are extremely painful. They hurt more than slashing wounds. You'll probably cause your attacker more immediate pain with a ballpoint pen than with a knife.

Another efficient weapon is a small, stiff hairbrush, which can be used to jab with the handle or to rake the bristles across the eyes.

I also suggest small canisters of pepper spray. Mace takes up to five seconds to work (a very long time in a combat situation); pepper sprays get nearly instantaneous results. They effect mucous membranes of the nose, throat, and eyes; they were developed to ward off bears and other large animals. Buy a spray with a range of fifteen to twenty feet, such as Bodyguard Pepper Defense Spray, manufactured by Bodyguard Industries. It's also worth noting that several companies market sprays that include red dyes that mark your assailant for identification purposes should he be apprehended by police.

Don't leave these weapons in your purse. If you don't carry your weapons in your hands, when you're attacked you won't have time to get to them. If you're walking on the street or headed for your car, clutch your ballpoint pen in your fist. To the average person, a pen doesn't look like a weapon. This advice is no less true for canisters of pepper spray. There are several effective sprays on the market that look like writing instruments.

Your main weapon, though, is not the ballpoint pen, the hairbrush, or the canister of chemical deterrent, but the simple element of surprise. Be smart and tough. Don't ever threaten an attacker with a chemical spray or any other weapon. This is a form of telegraphing. He may grab a convenient garbage can lid or a large box to block the spray or he may simply tackle you as you threaten him. The weapon is only as effective as the user. Don't ever pose with a weapon. If you pull it, use it as quickly and as efficiently as you can.

Should you use a chemical deterrent, it's important not to stand still after you spray your assailant. In some cases, chemical sprays have been known to enrage attackers; you can't afford to take the chance that a spray has completed the job for you. Either immediately leave the site of the hopefully thwarted attack before your would-be assailant has time to recover or, if it seems more practical, expediently follow through with appropriate hand strikes, kicks, or stomps.

How to Find a Good Martial Arts School

I want to tell you the truth as simply as I know how: Reading this or any other book won't teach you how to defend yourself. It can, however, point you in the right direction. You need to take what I've shown you and use it to find a good martial arts school. To be successful when you need to be, you must attend this school on a very regular basis. And you must work rigorously and diligently.

As I mentioned earlier, most martial arts schools don't teach the kind of techniques that you'll find useful. Be careful when you're shopping for self-defense instruction. There's a lot of chicanery in the martial arts and a considerable amount of well-intentioned, yet inept instruction. It's possible you won't find the school you need in your town. Do your shopping in person and not on the phone.

Many qualified as well as unqualified self-defense teachers require you to sign long-term contracts before you begin training. Don't obligate yourself before you know that this is the school for you. Ask the instructor if a discount or free trial training session is offered. The school you need will probably be one in which they don't concentrate on sport. If the school you're considering practices flashy kicks to the head, if they train with minimal or no contact, if students talk about their most recent successes at this or that karate tournament, and if the instructor tells you, "We also teach self-defense," this is definitely not the school for you.

Martial arts that tend to be taught as sport and that you'll likely find ineffective for personal defense include Tae Kwon Do, all tournament competition style karate, aikido, and Tang Soo Do. This doesn't mean that you can't find a good instructor who teaches one of these systems; it means that if you visit a school where one or more of these disciplines is taught, you'll want to observe that school carefully, with suspicion and with a trained, discerning eye.

The arts that you'll most likely find effective include kali and escrima (the Filipino martial arts), judo, kickboxing (which, unlike tournament karate, is practiced with all-out real world contact), hapkido, jujitsu, and some kung fu systems. The fact that a school teaches one or more of these arts (or claims to) doesn't mean that this is the school for you; it only means that the odds are better that this is a studio that correctly emphasizes realistic contact training for personal protection and street survival.

If you have doubts about the school you're looking at, keep this in mind: The school you *need* is a "stick your fingers in the eyes, knee 'em to the groin, head butt, bite the nose off kind of place."

Achieve and Maintain a Healthy Body and Mind

Bikram's Beginning Yoga Class by Bikram Choudhury
Sweat, strain, laugh, and do more for your health,
body, and general well-being than you ever imag-
ined possible as you take your Beginning Hatha
Yoga Class from Los Angeles' most famous yoga
teacher.

Bodymind by Ken Dychtwald, Ph.D.
This classic work integrates ancient knowledge with
modern body-analysis techniques of Reich, Fel-
denkrais, Perls, and Dychtwald's own intuitive ob-
servations.

Fitness Walking for Women
by Anne Kashiwa and James Rippe, M.D.
From the leading women's walking advocate and
the coauthor of the breakthrough book *Fitness Walking*, a walking program specifically tailored to
women's needs and concerns.

Jeanne Rose's Herbal Body Book by Jeanne Rose
An authoritative sourcebook for using herbs for a
healthy, natural, and beautiful body.

PMS: A Positive Program to Gain Control
by Stephanie DeGraff Bender
A psychologist and director of a PMS clinic shares
her successful program for treating the psychologi-
cal and physical symptoms of premenstrual syn-
drome.

PMS: Questions and Answers
by Stephanie DeGraff Bender
This important guide answers all the most fre-
quently asked questions about premenstrual syn-
drome.

History of Ideas on Woman by Rosemary Agonito
In a single volume—a collection of the primary
sources of Western civilization's attitudes toward
women, from Genesis and Plato, to Rousseau and
Freud—Agonito examines the evolution of women's
psychology, legal rights, virtues, and ethics.

*The Motherline: Every Woman's Journey to Find Her
Female Roots*
by Naomi Ruth Lowinsky, Ph.D.
Offering understanding and healing for the most
important relationship in a woman's life. Its wisdom
is timeless, like the motherline, from generation to
generation.

To Be a Woman: The Birth of the Conscious Feminine
edited by Connie Zweig
A striking collection of twenty-three original essays
by authorities in women's psychology.

No! No! No! by Kathy Long
Five-time world champion kickboxer Kathy Long
shows women how to defend themselves in almost
any situation. Illustrated with 100 black-and-white
photographs.

These books are available at your bookstore or wher-
ever books are sold, or, for your convenience, we'll
send them directly to you. Call 1-800-788-6262 or fill
out coupon on page 125 and send it to:

The Putnam Publishing Group
390 Murray Hill Parkway, Dept. B
East Rutherford, NJ 07073

About the Authors

Kathy Long is a five-time featherweight and bantamweight women's world kickboxing champion. In 1992, *Black Belt* magazine named Long "kickboxer of the year."

Long's martial arts background is extensive and multidimensional. She began studying aikido at age fifteen; at eighteen, she earned a black belt. At nineteen, she switched to *san soo* gung-fu. She was awarded her black belt in gung-fu when she was twenty-three. Long explains the basic differences between gung-fu and ring fighting. "Kickboxing is a sport," she says. "Inside the ring, although the opponent is trying to knock you out, if worse comes to worst, you can quit. In self-defense situations, there's so much more at stake. You can easily get raped or killed. Fighting, real fighting, is about sticking your fingers in people's eyes, crushing groins, breaking knees; you bite, you claw, you reshape people's skeletons."

In 1991, Long was named "Woman of the Year" by the *Black Belt* magazine hall of fame and she was elected to the *Inside Kung-fu* magazine hall of fame, considered to be the most prestigious awards a martial artist can attain in the United States. She's the first person to be honored with both awards in the same year and the only martial artist to be named to the *Black Belt* hall of fame two consecutive years.

Long teaches self-defense, gung-fu, and kickboxing in southern California.

Davis Miller is a contributing editor at *Sport* magazine, which is the best-selling monthly sports periodical in North America. In addition to his work for *Sport*, Miller's fiction and nonfiction have appeared in *Esquire*, *Men's Journal*, *Gentlemen's Quarterly*, *Sports Illustrated*, the *Louisville Courier-Journal Magazine*, the *Washington Post Magazine*, the *Los Angeles Times*, and many other publications. He has also written a film documentary about Bruce Lee for Warner Brothers called *Curse of the Dragon*.

The Sunday Magazine Editors Association judged his story, "My Dinner with Ali," to be the best essay published in a newspaper magazine in the United States in 1989. That same year, he was named Writer of the Year by the American Association for the Improvement of Boxing.

Miller lives in Winston-Salem, North Carolina. He is at work on a nonfiction novel about his unusual friendship with Muhammad Ali.

Bikram's Beginning Yoga Class	874-77082-3	$12.95
Bodymind	874-77375-X	$10.95
Fitness Walking for Women	399-51407-4	$ 9.95
Jeanne Rose's Herbal Body Book	399-50790-6	$10.95
PMS: A Positive Program to Gain Control	399-51758-8	$ 8.95
PMS: Questions and Answers	399-51759-6	$ 5.95
History of Ideas on Woman	399-50379-X	$11.95
The Motherline	874-77732-1	$12.95
To Be a Woman	399-77561-2	$12.95

Subtotal $_____

Postage and Handling* $_____

Sales Tax (CA, NJ, NY, PA) $_____

Total Amount Due $_____

Payable in U.S. funds (no cash orders accepted). $15.00 minimum for credit card orders.

* Postage and handling: $2.50 for 1 book, 75¢ for each additional book up to a maximum of $6.25.

Enclosed is my ☐ check ☐ money order
Please charge my ☐ Visa ☐ Mastercard ☐ American Express

Card # _____ Expiration Date _____

Signature as on charge card _____

Name _____

Address _____

City _____ State _____ Zip _____

Please allow six weeks for delivery. Prices subject to change without notice.

Source Key 63